HYPERTENSION BOOK GUIDE.

Ultimate Solutions to hypertension or blood pressure.

By Linda J Franklin

TABLE OF CONTENT

Chapter 1: Blood pressure or hypertension definition

Chapter 2: Types of Hypertension

Chapter 3: Hypertension in children

Chapter 4:Lowering blood pressure at home

Chapter 5: things to consume naturally to reduce blood pressure

Chapter 1: Blood pressure or hypertension definition

The pressure of your blood in your circulatory system is known as your blood pressure. Systolic blood pressure over diastolic blood pressure is used to measure blood pressure. Systolic blood pressure measures the force your blood applies to the walls of your arteries when your heart contracts and diastolic blood pressure measures the force your blood applies to the walls of your arteries when your heart is at rest. A systolic measurement of less than 120 mmHg and a diastolic value of less than 80 mmHg is considered normal blood pressure.

Although raised systolic or diastolic blood pressure alone may be used to diagnose high blood pressure or hypertension, elevated systolic or diastolic blood pressure is often given greater attention as a risk factor for cardiovascular disease.

Effects of high blood pressure on one's health (Hypertension)

Beyond cardiac disease, high blood pressure has detrimental effects on health.

the heart and arteries

Damage to your arteries and heart top the list of adverse health outcomes brought on by hypertension. Blood pressure in your arteries rises with hypertension, which may lead to aneurysms, damaged and restricted arteries, and an increase in blood pressure.

Atherosclerosis/narrowing of the arteries: Hypertension weakens the elasticity of your arteries' inner lining cells, which reduces blood flow throughout your body.Aneurysm: An aneurysm is a bulge that develops when pressure from blood flowing through a weak artery causes a wall portion to grow. Although aneurysms may develop in any artery in your body, they most often occur in your aorta (the largest artery in your body). A burst aneurysm may result in fatal internal bleeding.

Uncontrolled blood pressure may harm your heart by causing heart failure, an enlarged left ventricle, and coronary artery disease.

Narrowing of the blood arteries that feed blood to your heart is known as coronary artery disease.

Left heart enlargement: High blood pressure forces your heart to pump blood throughout your body more forcefully than is required. As a consequence, your left ventricle starts to thicken, which reduces its capacity to pump blood to the rest of the body. With this illness, there is an increased risk of heart attack and heart failure.

Heart failure: When your heart is under stress from high blood pressure, it starts to weaken, wear out, and fail.

In addition to dementia, stroke, and transient ischemic attack (TIA), cerebral hypertension may potentially harm your brain.

A transient ischaemic attack (TIA) is a brief, intermittent disturbance of your brain's blood flow that is often brought on by artery hardening or a blood clot.

More serious than a TIA, a stroke happens when a portion of your brain is deprived of oxygen and nutrients, which causes brain cells to degenerate. Blood clots or restricted, leaky, or burst blood arteries may be the reason for this.

Vascular dementia: Narrowing and blockage of arteries that carry blood to the brain may cause dementia.

Blood pressing against blood vessel walls is measured by blood pressure. Blood is pumped from the heart into blood arteries, where it travels throughout the body. High blood pressure, also known as hypertension, is harmful because it makes the heart work harder to pump blood to the body and increases the risk of heart failure, stroke, renal disease, atherosclerosis, and hardening of the arteries, or atherosclerosis.

This is how a blood pressure value is expressed: 120/80. It is pronounced, "120 over 80." Systolic refers to the top number, while diastolic refers to the bottom number. Ranges include:
Normal: 120 over 80 (120/80) or less
120–129/less than 80 elevated
Stage 1 hypertension: 130-139/80-89
The blood pressure of stage 2 is 140/90 or above.

Secondary hypertension is the term used to describe the disease when a direct cause of high blood pressure can be determined. Kidney illness is the most common cause of secondary hypertension. Additionally, tumors and other abnormalities that cause the tiny glands that sit on top of the kidneys, the adrenal glands, to emit excessive quantities of the hormones that raise blood pressure may result in hypertension. Pregnancy, the use of blood pressure-raising medicines, and birth control pills, particularly those that include estrogen, may all raise blood pressure.

people that have high blood pressure in their families
Smokers
African-Americans
expecting mothers
female users of birth control tablets
Overweight or obese individuals above the age of 35
People who are inactive People who consume excessive amounts of alcohol
those who consume excessive amounts of salty or fatty meals
Those who suffer from sleep apnea

Most of the time, it's unclear what causes high blood pressure. However, several factors might raise your risk.

High blood pressure has many known reasons.

High blood pressure results from an underlying medical problem or from taking a specific medication in around 1 in 20 instances.

The following medical problems may result in high blood pressure:

diabetes, chronic kidney infections, and kidney disease

Obstructive sleep apnoea occurs when the throat's muscles relax and constrict when a person is sleeping, preventing them from breathing normally.

acromegaly, Cushing's syndrome, hyperaldosteronism, glomerulonephritis, damage to the small filters within the kidneys, constriction of the arteries feeding the kidneys, and hormone issues such as hyperaldosteronism, hyperthyroidism, and pheochromocytoma.

lupus is an illness when the immune system affects the skin, joints, and organs of the body.

Skin that is thickened and occasionally has issues with organs and blood vessels is a symptom of the disorder scleroderma.

The following medications may raise your blood pressure:

steroids and the contraceptive pill

NSAIDs, or non-steroidal anti-inflammatory medications, include ibuprofen and naproxen.

certain prescription cough and cold medications

various herbal medicines, especially those that include licorice, and some illicit substances, such cocaine and amphetamines

Several SSNRIs, including venlafaxine, are selective serotonin-noradrenaline reuptake inhibitors (SSNRI) antidepressants.

In these circumstances, stopping the medication or substance use may cause your blood pressure to return to normal.

Chapter 2: Types of Hypertension

Younger adults with untreated hypertension are more likely to have kidney and brain damage, arterial hardening, and an increased risk of stroke.

The phrase "the silent killer" refers to high blood pressure.
Its silence often causes health issues in adolescents and young adults, which are then disregarded by physicians.
However, not treating the illness might have negative effects.
Being overweight and having a longer lifespan are two key lifestyle characteristics that are often linked to this high prevalence.
The likelihood of developing it might potentially reach up to 90%, according to some studies.

This isn't always the case with younger people, regardless of how careful physicians are in treating the illness in middle-aged and older people.

According to research published in the journal Postgraduate Medicine, "Active persons, especially the young and athletes, are considered as free of disorders such as hypertension."

However, the authors of the research noted that the increasing incidence of age-related risk factors, such as obesity, diabetes mellitus, and renal illness, increases the likelihood that younger persons may acquire hypertension.

Young individuals with high blood pressure, especially those with ISH, are often thought of as anomalies that will go away on their own.

Since it sometimes appears in high school athletes, it is even seen as a symbol of a strong heart.

Systolic blood pressure values should be 120/80 to be considered normal (diastolic).

Any value of 140/90 or above indicates hypertension.

Only the top (systolic) value is high in the case of ISH, whereas the bottom number is within a normal range.

"Young persons with increased blood pressure," said Vongpatanasin to Healthline, "even those with only a high systolic number, but a normal diastolic number may have an unusually stiff aorta, which should not be overlooked." They should closely monitor their health and consult with their primary care providers to determine if it requires treatment.

Adapting your way of life may be helpful. Through a mix of medication and lifestyle adjustments, hypertension is very curable.

One of the best strategies to reduce blood pressure is to modify eating and exercise routines.

Vongpatanasin advises eating meals that are high in fruits and vegetables.

Limiting salt consumption is essential for keeping blood pressure at a healthy level.

"I know that if I decrease your salt consumption in half, it lowers blood pressure," the doctor said, citing seven or eight different sorts of research that all point to the importance of salt.

According to experts, the current standard of treatment can no longer be treating the problem untreated in young people.

"It is unlikely that this situation will improve. It will grow worse, Vongpatanasin said.

staged hypertension

All blood pressure readings above 120/80 mm Hg are regarded as high under the revised 2017 standards.

Currently, blood pressure readings fall into the following categories:

elevated: less than 80 mm Hg in the diastolic and systolic blood pressure measurements
Stage 1: systolic or diastolic blood pressure between 80 and 89 millimeters of mercury
Stage 2: at least 140 mm Hg systolic or 90 mm Hg diastolic
More individuals who were previously classified as prehypertensive fall into the elevated group under the new categorization scheme.

According to the new recommendations, 46 percent of American adults are now considered to have high blood pressure.
If you have heart disease or other risk factors, such as diabetes and a family history of illness, treatment is advised at the high stage.
If your blood pressure measurement falls into the high range, talk to your doctor about what you can do to decrease it.

Secondary vs primary hypertension

early-stage hypertension
Essential hypertension is another name for primary hypertension. Adults who have hypertension often fall under this group.

Despite many studies, the exact etiology of hypertension is still unknown. Age, nutrition, lifestyle, and genetics are considered to have a role.
Smoking, excessive alcohol consumption, stress, being overweight, eating too much salt, and inactivity are all examples of lifestyle factors.
Your blood pressure and risk of consequences from hypertension may be reduced by making dietary and lifestyle changes.

Subsequent hypertension
When your hypertension has a known, perhaps treatable cause, it is said to be secondary hypertension.

The secondary kind of hypertension accounts for just 5 to 10 percent of cases.

Younger people are more prone to it. Secondary hypertension is thought to affect 30% of people with hypertension between the ages of 18 and 40.

The following are the underlying causes of secondary hypertension:
adrenal gland illness constriction of the arteries supplying blood to your kidneys negative effects of various drugs, such as birth control pills, diet supplements, stimulants, antidepressants, and some over-the-counter drugs
anomalies in the obstructive sleep apnea hormone
aberrant thyroid functions
narrowing of the aorta

Additional forms of hypertension
The following subtypes fall within the main or secondary hypertension categories:

unresponsive hypertension
idiopathic hypertension
one-off hypertension
stubborn hypertension
The term "resistant hypertension" refers to high blood pressure that is difficult to manage and calls for many drugs.
When your blood pressure continues to be higher than your treatment goal after using three different blood pressure-lowering drugs, including a diuretic, your hypertension is deemed resistant.

Resistant hypertension affects around 10%Trusted Source of individuals with high blood pressure.

Patients with resistant hypertension may also have secondary hypertension, for which no secondary reasons have been found, necessitating a search for secondary causes by their doctor.

The majority of patients with resistant hypertension may be effectively treated with a combination of medications or by identifying a secondary cause.

idiopathic hypertension
The phrase "malignant hypertension" refers to excessive blood pressure that harms your organs. There is an emergency here.
The most severe kind of hypertension, known as malignant hypertension, is characterized by various organ damage and increased blood pressure that is often >180 mm Hg systolic or >120-130 mm Hg diastolic.

Malignant hypertension is rare, with just 1 to 2 incidences per 100,000 people. In black populations, rates might be greater.

Malignant hypertension is a medical emergency that has to be treated right away. If you believe you may be experiencing a hypertensive crisis, get urgent emergency medical assistance.

isolated systolic hypertension
Systolic blood pressure above 140 mm Hg and diastolic pressure under 90 mm Hg are considered isolated systolic hypertension.
In elderly individuals, it is the most prevalent kind of hypertension. Isolated systolic hypertension affects around 15% of adults 60 years of age or older Trusted Source.
The arteries hardening with age is considered to be the reason.

Systolic hypertension that is isolated may also appear in younger persons. 2% to 8% of younger persons have isolated systolic hypertension, In young people aged 17 to 27, it is the most prevalent type of hypertension, according to a UK survey.

Younger and middle-aged adults with isolated systolic hypertension had a greater risk of stroke and heart attack than those with normal blood pressure, according to a large 2015 research with an average of 31 years of follow-up.

emergency hypertension
When your blood pressure unexpectedly climbs over 180/120 and you have symptoms as a result of this abrupt spike in blood pressure, you are experiencing a hypertensive emergency, also known as malignant hypertension. These consist of:

headache, shortness of breath, dizziness, chest discomfort, and altered vision
High blood pressure poses a danger to life since it may harm vital organs or result in consequences such as aortic dissection, aortic rupture, or brain hemorrhage.

If you believe you may be experiencing a hypertensive crisis, get urgent emergency medical assistance.

Only 1% to 3% of hypertensive patients are likely to have hypertensive crises throughout their lifetime. Take your blood pressure medicine as directed, and stay away from stimulant medications since they often lead to hypertensive emergencies.
heightened urgency
When your blood pressure is over 180/120 but you have no other symptoms, you are said to have hypertensive urgency.

The most common way to address hypertensive urgency is to change your medication schedule. To prevent a hypertensive emergency, it is crucial to address hypertensive urgency very away.
It's a dangerous illness, so if you have hypertension urgency, you should phone your doctor's office right away or get medical attention. Less than 1% of persons with hypertensive urgency are sent to a hospital, and few of them have negative repercussions.

WHITE COAT HIGH PRESSURE?
This phrase describes situations when your blood pressure may spike briefly due to being at a doctor's office or experiencing another stressful situation, such as being trapped in traffic.

This disorder has previously been determined to be benign. It has lately been linked to a higher risk of cardiovascular disease. People who have white coat hypertension often go on to develop hypertension.

Your doctor will often check your blood pressure in several situations over time before prescribing a prescription for hypertension. Any reading outside of range should be reviewed with your doctor since your diagnosis won't be based on just one reading.

You can prevent and treat high blood pressure, which is excellent news.

Monitor your blood pressure.
If you are in danger, a first approach is to routinely check your blood pressure. You may use a blood pressure monitoring kit at home or have your doctor do it in the office. You'll be able to determine if any blood pressure drugs or other treatments have an impact if you're taking them.

taking blood pressure readings
The pressure your heart generates as it beats forces blood through your circulatory system. Two values, expressed in millimeters of mercury, are used to calculate your blood pressure (mm Hg).

The pressure at which your blood is being pushed from your heart to your arteries is shown by the first (top) number. We refer to this as systolic blood pressure.
The pressure between beats of your heart is shown by the second (lower) number. We refer to this as diastolic blood pressure.
alterations in way of life

To avoid hypertension or to manage your hypertension, think about adopting lifestyle modifications. Exercise is very good in bringing down blood pressure.

The following adjustments may also be helpful:
not a smoker
consuming a balanced diet and limiting sugar and carbs
avoiding alcohol or using it sparingly while keeping a healthy weight
controlling your stress
eating more potassium and less salt
Medications on prescription
Your doctor could prescribe one or more prescription medicines to lower your blood pressure depending on your risk factors and degree of hypertension. Medication is always used in tandem with lifestyle changes.

Medication to reduce blood pressure comes in a variety of forms. They operate on several philosophies.

The finest medications for you may be discussed with your doctor. Finding the ideal mixture could take some time. Each person is unique.

It's crucial to take your medications as prescribed and to see your doctor often, particularly if your health or blood pressure seems to be changing.

controlling second-degree hypertension
Your doctor will treat the underlying disease first if your hypertension is related to another illness.

People with high blood pressure under the age of 30 are often suspicious of secondary hypertension.

Following are some indicators of secondary hypertension:

an abrupt increase in blood pressure that requires more than three medications to maintain hypertension under control signs and symptoms of thyroid disease, renal artery stenosis, and syphilis

Chapter 3: Hypertension in children

High blood pressure (hypertension) in children is blood pressure that is at or above the 95th percentile for children who are the same sex, age, and height as your child. There isn't a simple target range for high blood pressure in all children because what's considered normal changes as children grow. However, in teenagers, high blood pressure is defined the same as for adults: A blood pressure reading greater than or equal to 130/80 millimeters of mercury (mm Hg).

The younger a child is, the more likely it is that the high blood pressure is caused by a specific and identifiable medical condition. Older children can develop high blood pressure for the same reasons adults do — excess weight, poor nutrition, and lack of exercise.

Lifestyle changes, such as eating a heart-healthy diet low in salt (sodium) and exercising more, can help reduce high blood pressure in children. But for some children, medications may be necessary.

Symptoms
High blood pressure usually doesn't cause symptoms. However, signs and symptoms that might indicate a high blood pressure emergency (hypertensive crisis) include:

Headaches
Seizures
Vomiting
Chest pains
Fast, pounding, or fluttering heartbeat (palpitations)
Shortness of breath
If your child has any of these signs or symptoms, seek emergency medical care.

Your child's blood pressure should be checked during routine well-check appointments starting at age 3, and at every appointment, if your child is found to have high blood pressure.

If your child has a condition that can increase the risk of high blood pressure — including premature birth, low birth weight, congenital heart disease, and certain kidney problems — blood pressure checks might begin soon after birth.

If you're concerned about your child having a risk factor for high blood pressure, such as obesity, talk to your child's doctor.

Causes
High blood pressure in younger children is often related to other health conditions, such as heart defects, kidney disease, genetic conditions, or hormonal disorders. Older children — especially those who are

overweight — are more likely to have primary hypertension. This type of high blood pressure occurs on its own, without an underlying condition.

Your child's risk factors for high blood pressure depend on health conditions, genetics, and lifestyle factors.

Primary (essential) hypertension
Primary hypertension occurs on its own, without an identifiable cause. This type of high blood pressure occurs more often in children aged 6 and older. The risk factors for developing primary hypertension include:

Chronic kidney disease
Polycystic kidney disease
Heart problems, such as severe narrowing (coarctation) of the aorta
Adrenal disorders

Overactive thyroid (hyperthyroidism)

Narrowing of the artery to the kidney (renal artery stenosis)

Sleep disorders, especially obstructive sleep apnea

Certain drugs and medications, including those used to relieve a stuffy nose (decongestants), stimulants used to treat attention-deficit/hyperactivity disorder (ADHD), caffeine, nonsteroidal anti-inflammatory drugs (NSAIDs), and steroids

Cocaine, methamphetamine, and similar drugs

Complications

Children who have high blood pressure are likely to continue to have high blood pressure as adults unless they begin treatment.

If your child's high blood pressure continues into adulthood, your child could be at risk of:

Stroke

Heart attack

Heart failure

Kidney disease

Prevention

High blood pressure can be prevented in children by making the same lifestyle changes that can help treat it — controlling your child's weight, providing a healthy diet low in salt (sodium), and encouraging your child to exercise.

High blood pressure caused by another condition can sometimes be controlled, or even prevented, by managing the condition that's causing it.

Chapter 4:Lowering blood pressure at home

1. Be more active and more active
Aerobic and weight training may considerably reduce blood pressure, particularly for males, according to a meta-analysis of 65 research.

In a 2013 research, inactive older individuals who engaged in aerobic exercise training had an average reduction in systolic and diastolic blood pressure of 3.9 and 4.5 percent, respectively. These outcomes are comparable to those of various blood pressure medicines.

Your heart grows stronger and pumps less forcefully as you routinely raise your heart and breathing rates. This decreases your blood pressure and relieves pressure on your arteries.

If it's hard to find 40 minutes at once, breaking it up into three or four 10- to 15-minute chunks throughout the day could still be beneficial.

It's not necessary to run marathons, however. You may increase your activity level by doing the following:

utilizing the stairs, walking rather than driving, doing laundry, gardening, going on a bike trip, or participating in a team sport Just be consistent and build up to at least 30 minutes of moderate exercise each day.

Tai chi is one instance of a modest exercise that may have significant effects. In comparison to no exercise at all, a 2017 assessment on the effects of tai chi and high blood pressure found an average overall decline in systolic blood pressure of 15.6 mm Hg and a diastolic blood pressure drop of 10.7 mm Hg.

Several combinations of exercise may reduce blood pressure, according to 2014 research on the topic.

These drills consist of:
Walking 10,000 steps a day, aerobic exercise, strength training, high-intensity interval training, and brief bursts of exercise throughout the day.
There are still advantages to even little physical exercise, particularly for older persons, according to ongoing research.

2. If you are overweight, lose weight.
Losing 5 to 10 pounds might lower your blood pressure if you are overweight. Additionally, you'll reduce your likelihood of developing other medical issues.

According to a review of multiple research, weight reduction regimens typically lower blood pressure by 3.2 mm Hg diastolic and 4.5 mm Hg systolic.

3. Consume less refined carbs and sugars
Numerous studies have shown that limiting sugar and processed carbs may aid in weight loss and blood pressure reduction.
According to 2014 research, sugar, particularly fructose, may raise blood pressure more than salt. Sugar elevated blood pressure by 6.9 mm Hg systolic and 5.6 mm Hg diastolic in studies that lasted at least 8 weeks.

According to a 2020 research comparing many common diets, low-carb and low-fat diets reduced systolic blood pressure by 3 mm Hg and diastolic blood pressure by an average of 5 mm Hg in adults who were overweight or obese after six month.

Because you're eating more protein and fat on a low-carb, low-sugar diet, you feel satiated for longer.

4. Consume a lot of potassium and little sodium.

Salt reduction and potassium dietary supplementation may both reduce blood pressure.

Potassium benefits your body in two ways: it lowers the impact of salt on your system and reduces blood vessel stress. However, potassium-rich diets may be dangerous to those who have a renal illness, so consult your doctor before consuming more potassium.

It is simple to consume extra potassium. Naturally rich in potassium foods abound. To name a few:

Low-fat dairy products like milk and yogurt, fish, and fruits like bananas, apricots, avocados, and oranges as well as vegetables like potatoes, tomatoes, spinach, and sweet potatoes.

Keep in mind that everyone reacts to salt differently. Some individuals have salt sensitivity, which causes their blood pressure to rise when they consume more salt. Others don't react to salt. They may consume a lot of salt and eliminate it in their urine without their blood pressure increasing.

The DASH (Dietary Approaches to Stop Hypertension) diet is advised by the National Institutes of Health as a means of lowering salt consumption. The DASH diet focuses on:

foods low in sodium
veggies and fruits, low-fat dairy, and whole grains
fewer sweets, red meats, and poultry, poultry, and beans

5. Consume less processed foods
Your salt shaker at home does not provide the majority of the excess salt in your diet that comes from processed meals and foods

from restaurants. Products with a lot of salt are common:

cold cuts
tins of soup
pizza\schips
additional prepared foods
To make up for the loss of fat, "low fat" foods often have high salt and sugar content. Food tastes better and helps you feel full when it is fatty.

You may consume less salt, sugar, and refined carbs by limiting your intake of processed foods, or even better, by eliminating them from your diet. Lower blood pressure may be the outcome of all of these.

Make reading nutrition labels a habit. 5 percent or less of the salt listed on a product label is regarded as low by the Food and Drug Administration (FDA), whereas 20 percent or more is regarded as excessive.

Six. Quit smoking.
Although it might be challenging, giving up smoking is beneficial for your general health. The sudden but transient rise in blood pressure and heart rate brought on by smoking.

Through blood vessel wall deterioration, inflammation, and artery constriction over time, tobacco's compounds may raise blood pressure. Higher blood pressure is a result of the hardened arteries.

Even when exposed to secondhand smoke, the compounds in tobacco may hurt your blood vessels.
According to research, nonsmokers who had access to smoke-free workplaces, pubs, and eateries had lower blood pressure than nonsmokers who lived in locations without any laws governing smoke-free environments.

7. Lower excessive tension

We are at a challenging period. Stress is a result of pressures on the job and at home, as well as domestic and international affairs. Your health and blood pressure depend on you finding strategies to lessen your stress.

Discover what works for you among the many effective stress-relieving techniques available. Do some deep breathing exercises, go on a stroll, pick up a book, or watch a comedy.

It has also been shown that regular music listening lowers systolic blood pressure.

Regular sauna usage decreased the risk of dying from heart-related causes, according to 20-year research.

Additionally, short research conducted in 2015 found that acupuncture may reduce both systolic and diastolic blood pressure.

8. Try yoga or meditation.

Stress reduction techniques that have been used and researched for a long time include transcendental meditation and mindfulness. Yoga, which often incorporates breathing exercises, posture corrections, and meditation methods, may also help lower blood pressure and stress levels.

When compared to those who didn't exercise, 2013 research on yoga and blood pressure reported an average blood pressure decline of 3.62 mm Hg diastolic and 4.17 mm Hg systolic.

Studies of yoga practices found that those that incorporated breath control, postures, and meditation were almost twice as successful as those that did not.

9. Consume some chocolate.
Chocolate lovers: There is evidence that dark chocolate may reduce blood pressure.

But 60 to 70 percent cacao should be present in the dark chocolate. One to two squares of dark chocolate per day may help decrease the risk of heart disease by reducing blood pressure and inflammation, according to a review of research on the subject.

The flavonoids found in chocolate with greater cocoa solids are considered to be responsible for the advantages. Your blood arteries may dilate or expand with the aid of flavonoids.

10. Examine these healing plants.
Many civilizations have utilized herbal remedies for a long time to cure a range of illnesses.

Even certain herbs have the potential to reduce blood pressure. To determine the dosages and elements in the herbs that are most effective, additional study is necessary.

Before using herbal supplements, always consult your physician or pharmacist. They could conflict with your prescription drugs.

Various civilizations throughout the globe utilize the following limited list of plants and herbs to decrease blood pressure:

bean black (Castanospermum australe)
feline claw (Uncaria rhynchophylla)
carrot juice (Apium graveolens)
Chinese huckleberry (Crataegus pinnatifida)
gigantic dodder of ginger (Cuscuta reflexa)
Native Plants (blond psyllium)
coastal pine bark (Pinus pinaster)
Fluvial lily (Crinum glaucum)
roselle (Hibiscus sabdariffa)
tahini oil (Sesamum indicum)
tomato juice (Lycopersicon esculentum)
tea (Camellia sinensis), particularly oolong and green tea tree bark (Musanga cecropioides)

11. Ensure that you receive enough restorative sleep.
When you sleep, your blood pressure normally drops. Your blood pressure may be impacted by poor sleep.

People who lack sleep, particularly those in their middle years, are more likely to develop high blood pressure.

It might be difficult for some individuals to obtain a decent night's sleep. Here are a few strategies to aid in a pleasant night's sleep:

Consider creating a consistent sleep pattern.
Before going to bed, relax.
Engage in daytime exercise.
Avoid taking naps throughout the day.
Make sure your bedroom is cozy.
A regular sleep pattern of fewer than 7 hours per night or more than 9 hours per night was linked to an elevated risk of high blood pressure, according to the 2010 national Sleep Heart Health Study.

Regularly getting less than 5 hours of sleep every night was associated with a considerable long-term risk of high blood pressure.

12. Consume garlic or supplement with garlic extract
Both raw and extracted garlic is often used to decrease blood pressure.

According to a meta-analysis, garlic supplements may lower systolic blood pressure by up to 5 mm Hg and diastolic blood pressure by up to 2.5 mm Hg in persons with high blood pressure.

A 2009 clinical investigation found that time-release garlic extract preparations may lower blood pressure more than conventional garlic powder pills.

13. Consume wholesome, high-protein meals

People who consumed more protein had a decreased risk of high blood pressure, according to long-term research that was completed in 2014. Compared to those on a low protein diet, individuals who consumed an average of 100 grams of protein per day had a 40% decreased chance of developing high blood pressure.

Additionally, those who increased their intake of normal fiber saw a risk decrease of up to 60%.

A high-protein diet may not be suitable for everyone, however. Kidney disease sufferers may need to exercise care. It's better to consult your physician.

On the majority of diet plans, getting 100 grams of protein per day is not too difficult.

foods high in protein include:

seafood, such as canned tuna or salmon, and eggs
beef, kidney beans, lentils, nuts, or nut butter, such as peanut butter, poultry, such as chicken breast, beans, and legumes, such as lentils and kidney beans.
cheddar-style chickpea cheese
While a 3.5-ounce meal of chicken breast may have 30 grams of protein, a 3.5-ounce dish of salmon may have up to 22 grams.

For vegetarian choices, most varieties of beans include 7 to 10 grams of protein per half-cup meal. Eight grams would be present in two tablespoons of peanut butter.
Take these blood pressure-lowering vitamins,
These commonly accessible substances have shown potential in decreasing blood pressure:

Polyunsaturated fatty acid omega-3

There are several advantages of including fish oil or omega-3 polyunsaturated fatty acids in your diet.

A meta-analysis of fish oil and blood pressure revealed a mean 4.5 mm Hg systolic and 3.0 mm Hg diastolic decrease in people with high blood pressure.

Yogurt protein
This milk-derived protein complex could also improve several other bodily functions in addition to potentially decreasing blood pressure.
Magnesium
Higher blood pressure is associated with magnesium shortage. A meta-analysis found that taking more magnesium led to a little drop in blood pressure.
Citrulline
L-citrulline, taken orally, is a precursor to L-arginine, a protein building block that may reduce blood pressure.

15. Consume less booze

Even if you're in good health, alcohol may cause your blood pressure to rise.

It's crucial to drink responsibly. A 2006 research found that drinking alcohol might cause your blood pressure to rise by 1 mm Hg for every 10 grams consumed. A typical beverage has 14 grams of alcohol.

What does a typical drink consist of? 1.5 ounces of distilled liquor, 5 ounces of wine, or one 12-ounce lager.

Up to one drink per day for women and up to two drinks per day for males is considered moderate drinking.

According to a study, even while consuming more than 30 grams of alcohol may initially reduce blood pressure, after 13 hours or longer, systolic and diastolic blood pressure rose by 3.7 mm Hg and 2.4 mm Hg, respectively.

16. Take into account consuming less caffeine

Although it temporarily increases blood pressure, caffeine does so.

In a 2017 research, drinking 32 ounces of either a caffeinated beverage or an energy drink caused the systolic blood pressure of 18 individuals to rise for two hours. The subjects who had a caffeinated beverage then saw a quicker decline in blood pressure.

Caffeine may affect some individuals differently than others. If you're sensitive to caffeine, you may wish to drink less coffee or switch to decaffeinated coffee.

There has been a lot of research on caffeine, including its advantages in terms of health. The decision to make cuts is influenced by a variety of unique elements.

Prior research found that if your blood pressure is already high, coffee would have a bigger influence on boosting it. However, this same study recommended more investigation of the issue.

17. Use prescription drugs
Your doctor could suggest prescription medicines if your blood pressure is high or doesn't drop after making these lifestyle modifications.

They are effective and will enhance your long-term results, particularly if you have other risk factors. Finding the ideal pharmaceutical mix, however, might take some time.

Discuss potential drugs and which ones would be most effective for you with your doctor.

Chapter 5: things to consume naturally to reduce blood pressure

1.Berries Antioxidant substances called anthocyanins, a kind of flavonoid, are found in strawberries and blueberries.

In a previous study, the researchers examined data for more than 34,000 hypertensive patients over 14 years. those who consume the most anthocyanins.

However, a few specialists

According to a reliable source, there is insufficient proof that blueberries lower blood pressure.

Berry enjoyment:

Following meals, have them as a sweet treat or snack.

Sprinkle them on morning porridge and smoothies.

A cup of fresh, frozen, or half a cup of dried blueberries constitutes one serving of blueberries. Around 7 strawberries make a dish of strawberries.

1. Peaches

Potassium, which is present in bananas, may help control hypertension. 422 milligrams (mg) of potassium may be found in one medium banana, a Trusted Source of potassium.

The American Heart Association (AHA)Trusted Source claims that potassium counteracts the negative effects of sodium and eases stress in the blood vessel walls.

Males should try to get 3,400 mgTrusted Source of potassium daily, while females should consume 2,600 mg, according to the Office of Dietary Supplements.

Other foods high in potassium include:

acorn squash, potatoes, lentils, prunes, and apricots

Before increasing their potassium consumption, individuals with renal illness should speak with a doctor since too much potassium may be dangerous.

One giant banana, one cup of sliced bananas, or two-thirds of a cup of mashed banana would constitute a serving.

3. Beets

Because beet juice includes dietary nitrate, it may lower blood pressure both temporarily and permanently. Blood pressure was lowered in hypertensive individuals who consumed 250 milliliters (ml), or approximately 1 cup, of red beet juice every day for four weeks. Over 24 hours, the researchers observed an average drop in blood pressure of 7.7/5.2 millimeters of mercury (mm Hg).

Useful hints include:

daily consumption of one glass of beet juice
Beets are added to salads.
beet preparation as a side dish

A serving of beets is around one cup, which is equivalent to two small or one big beet.

4. Kiwis
According to a 2015 research by Trusted Source, kiwis may help control slightly elevated blood pressure if eaten regularly.
For 8 weeks, those who had 3 kiwis daily exhibited a greater decrease in systolic and diastolic blood pressure than those who consumed 1 apple daily. The authors of the research speculate that this could be because of the bioactive compounds in kiwis.

Kiwis contain a lot of vitamin C. People's blood pressure levels significantly decreased after taking 500 mg of vitamin C daily for roughly 8 weeks.
Kiwis are simple to include in smoothies or meals. 2-3 kiwifruits or one cup of kiwi constitute one serving.
Fifth, Watermelon

Citrulline is an amino acid that may be found in watermelon.

Citrulline is transformed by the body into arginine, which aids in the production of nitric oxide, a gas that relaxes blood vessels and promotes flexibility in arteries. Blood flow is improved as a result of these actions, which may decrease high blood pressure.

Adults with obesity and moderate or prehypertension in an earlier trial consumed a watermelon extract supplemented with 6 grams (g) of L-citrulline/L-arginine.

The subjects saw a decrease in blood pressure in their ankles and brachial arteries after 6 weeks. The primary artery in the upper arm is the brachial artery.
Although the guys did, the ladies who drank watermelon juice did not report a spike in blood pressure after exercise.

Watermelon may be consumed by people:

as juice in soups, salads, smoothies, and chilled watermelon dishes.
A serving of watermelon is one slice or about a cup of diced fruit.

6. Oats
Beta-glucan, a kind of fiber found in oats, may offer advantages.
Blood pressure information from a reliable source.

In hypertensive rats, beta-glucan and avenanthramide C, both contained in oats, were shown to lower levels of malondialdehyde, a sign of oxidative stress. These findings imply that components found in oats may help lower blood pressure and safeguard the heart in other ways.

Among the ways to consume oats are:

utilizing rolled oats in place of breadcrumbs to lend texture to burger patties and dusting them over yogurt desserts, eating a bowl of oatmeal for breakfast.

8. Green leafy veggies

The high nitrate content of leafy green vegetables helps control blood pressure.

Some analysis

According to a reliable source, consuming at least 1 cup of leafy green vegetables each day may decrease blood pressure and minimize the chance of developing cardiovascular disease.

Leafy greens include, for instance:
lettuce with collard greens
mustard greens, kale
spinach
Geneva chard
To acquire your recommended daily allowance of green vegetables, you can:

Add spinach to stews and curries.
as a side dish, sauté Swiss chard with garlic.
Bake some kale chips.
Two cups of fresh spinach constitute one serving. 1 cup is the serving size for raw cabbage.

Garlic 9.
Many of garlic's antibacterial and antifungal activities may be attributed to allicin, the major active component.

According to a reliable source, Kyolic garlic in particular, and garlic in general, might lessen:
arterial stiffness, cholesterol, and blood pressure
Stir-fries, soups, and omelets are just a few of the savory dishes that garlic may improve in taste. It may also be used as a seasoning in place of salt.
Ten. Fermented foods

Probiotics are good bacteria that are abundant in fermented foods and may help control blood pressure.

Data on 11,566 Korean people who are 50 years of age or older were examined by researchers. The findings imply that menopausal women who consumed fermented soy foods had a decreased incidence of hypertension. For males, that didn't seem to be the case, however.

Experts urge consumers to restrict their salt consumption since it raises blood pressure risk. Despite the high sodium content, 2017 research did not discover that consuming salt-fermented veggies increased the risk of high blood pressure.

Probiotics' positive effects on blood pressure seemed to be greater when participants consumed:
a variety of probiotic bacterial species

taking probiotics daily for at least 100 billion colony-forming units for more than 8 weeks

Included among the fermented items in your diet are:

miso tempeh kombucha apple cider vinegar kimchi

Supplements with probiotics are still another choice.

11. Pulses and other legumes

Lentils are a good source of protein and fiber, and according to experts' trusted Sources, they may help hypertensive people's blood vessels.

Rat diets high in pulses were examined by the authors of an earlier study trusted Source. 30% of the rats' diets consisted of pulses such as beans, peas, lentils, and chickpeas. Consuming pulses seems to lower blood pressure and cholesterol levels.

Lentils may be used in a variety of ways, such as:
as a replacement for minced beef, to give heft to salads, and as a foundation for stews and soups

12. Organic yogurt
Fermented dairy products include yogurt.
The individuals with high blood pressure who ate more yogurt had reduced systolic and arterial blood pressure compared to the non-participants.
How to enjoy plain yogurt:

Use it in place of cream over fruit and sweets, or add one tablespoon to a side dish of stew or curry with diced cucumber, mint, and garlic.
For breakfast, pour it over a mixture of oats, nuts, and dried fruit. Pomegranates
Antioxidants and other components found in pomegranates may assist to prevent atherosclerosis and high blood pressure.

There is proof that consuming 1 cup of pomegranate juice every day for 28 days will reduce high blood pressure temporarily.
Pomegranates may be eaten whole or juiced by consumers. Make sure there is no added sugar when purchasing premade pomegranate juice.

Cinnamon, 14.
cinnamon may help lower blood pressure. The researchers discovered that persons with a body mass index of 30 or above had lower blood pressure after taking up to 2 g of cinnamon daily for at least eight weeks.

Cinnamon may be added to the diet in the following ways:
Oatmeal may be made using it in place of sugar.
Add it to recently cut fruit.
Including it in smoothies. Numerous research has shown that consuming a variety of nuts may assist in controlling hypertension.

The endothelial function seems to be enhanced in walnuts, hazelnuts, and pistachios. This may help blood pressure and heart health.

Choose unsalted nuts, and:
eat them simply as a snack
Add them to salads; make pestos with them, and use them in major courses like nut roast
If a person has a nut allergy, they shouldn't eat nuts.

Citrus fruits 16
Hesperidin, an antioxidant found in citrus fruits, may be good for heart health.
According to the findings, hesperidin has a role in the lowering of systolic blood pressure that may be achieved by frequently ingesting orange juice.

Citrus fruit may be consumed by people:
as beverages, such as producing orange juice or squeezing entire lemons into the water, or in fruit salads, like using the lemon juice

from oranges and grapefruit to flavor salads instead of salt.

17. fatty fish

According to the AHA, eating two servings (each weighing three ounces, or oz) each week of oily fish may reduce the risk of cardiovascular disease.

Additionally, eating oily fish may help decrease blood pressure, according to a research-validated source. In 2016, after taking 0.7 g of eicosapentaenoic acid and docosahexaenoic acid fish oil supplements daily for 8 weeks, patients with high systolic blood pressure had considerable reductions in their readings.

Oily fish examples include:

Sardines, mackerel, albacore tuna, and anchovies
People should review the most recent Food and Drug Administration (FDA)Trusted Source recommendations since certain fish

contain mercury. Additionally, they may check this webpage to see whether fish are now sustainable.

18. Tomatillosulfonate
Lycopene, an antioxidant found in tomatoes, may be good for heart health.

Foods to avoid
While certain meals help lower blood pressure, others might raise the risk of the disorder.
According to salt studies, a little reduction in salt consumption for four or more weeks may considerably lower blood pressure.

One teaspoon (5.75 g) of salt, or 2.3 trusted sources of sodium, is the USDA's suggested daily upper limit.

Caffeine
Results of a review from 2011
According to a reliable source, taking 200 to 300 mg of caffeine may raise systolic blood

pressure by 5.7 mm Hg and diastolic blood pressure by 8.1 mm Hg within an hour. More than three hours passed before the blood pressure began to climb.

Alcohol

Alcohol use regularly considerably raises the risk of high blood pressure. Even modest drinking may have this effect on females. According to a 2021 evaluation by Trusted Source, there is no proof that low to moderate consumption provides any advantages for heart disease or hypertension.

keeping alcohol intake to no more than 2 drinks per day for men and 1 drink per day for women. 12 oz of beer, 5 oz of wine, or 1-1.5 oz of hard liquor constitute one serving of an alcoholic beverage, according to Trusted Source.

packaged food

Processed meals often include more salt and unhealthy fats. People who consume a lot of

processed foods are more likely to develop
high blood pressure.